Kidney Disease Diet For Seniors On Stage 3

Comprehensive Dietary Guidance for Maintaining Renal Function and Overall Wellbeing in Older Adults with Moderately Impaired Nephric Function.

Anita Hulsey

Copyright © 2024 [Anita Hulsey]

All rights reserved. No part of this publication may be reproduced, distributed, or transmitted in any form or by any means, including photocopying, recording, or other electronic or mechanical methods, without the prior written permission of the publisher, except in the case of brief quotations embodied in critical reviews and certain other noncommercial uses permitted by copyright law.

INTRODUCTION

Simon, a 72-year-old retiree, has been carefully managing his moderately impaired kidney function for several years now. As he navigates the complexities of stage 3 chronic kidney disease, Simon is determined to maintain his overall health and wellbeing through strategic dietary choices.

Recognizing the crucial role that proper nutrition plays in supporting renal function and preventing further decline, Simon has sought out the latest dietary guidance tailored for individuals with moderately compromised kidney health. This comprehensive overview aims to provide Simon and others like him with the essential information they need to make informed decisions about their dietary intake and optimize their kidney function.

By following the guidance outlined in this document, Simon hopes to preserve his remaining kidney function, manage any associated symptoms, and enjoy a fulfilling retirement without the burden of rapidly progressing kidney disease. As an active participant in his own care, Simon is eager to take control of his health and maintain his quality of life.

This dietary guidance is designed to empower individuals with moderately impaired kidney function, like Simon, to make mindful choices about their nutrient intake, manage their condition, and ultimately, support their overall wellbeing. With the right dietary strategies, Simon and others in his position can take proactive steps towards preserving their renal health and living their best lives.

Table of Contents

Recipe 1:
Classic Oatmeal with Mixed Berries and Almonds
Blueberry Walnut Oatmeal
Recipe 3:
Strawberry Pecan Oatmeal
Recipe 4:
Raspberry Hazelnut Oatmeal
Recipe 1:
Classic Vegetable Frittata
Recipe 2:
Broccoli and Mushroom Frittata
Recipe 3:
Zucchini and Tomato Frittata
Recipe 4:
Spinach and Red Pepper Frittata
Recipe 1:
Classic Whole Wheat Toast with Avocado and Poached Egg
Recipe 2:
Whole Wheat Toast with Avocado, Poached Egg, and Cherry Tomatoes
Recipe 3:
Whole Wheat Toast with Avocado, Poached Egg, and Feta Cheese
Recipe 4:
Whole Wheat Toast with Avocado, Poached

Egg, and Smoked Salmon

Recipe 1: Classic Greek Yogurt with Granola and Kiwi

Recipe 2:
Greek Yogurt with Granola, Kiwi, and Berries

Recipe 3:
Greek Yogurt with Granola, Kiwi, and Almonds

Recipe 4:
Greek Yogurt with Granola, Kiwi, and Coconut

Recipe 1:
Classic Grilled Salmon with Roasted Vegetables

Recipe 2:
Grilled Salmon with Roasted Brussels Sprouts and Sweet Potatoes

Recipe 3:
Grilled Salmon with Roasted Asparagus and Cherry Tomatoes

Recipe 4:
Grilled Salmon with Roasted Broccoli and Red Bell Peppers

Recipe 1:
Classic Quinoa and Spinach Salad with Feta

Recipe 2:
Quinoa and Spinach Salad with Feta and Cherry Tomatoes

Recipe 3:
Quinoa and Spinach Salad with Feta and

Avocado

Recipe 4:

Quinoa and Spinach Salad with Feta and Cucumbers

Recipe 1:

Classic Lentil and Sweet Potato Soup

Recipe 2:

Lentil and Sweet Potato Soup with Spinach

Recipe 3:

Lentil and Sweet Potato Soup with Coconut Milk

Recipe 4:

Spicy Lentil and Sweet Potato Soup

Recipe 1: Classic Brown Rice Bowl with Sautéed Shrimp and Broccoli

Recipe 2:

Brown Rice Bowl with Sautéed Shrimp, Broccoli, and Carrots

Recipe 3:

Brown Rice Bowl with Sautéed Shrimp, Broccoli, and Bell Peppers

Recipe 4:

Brown Rice Bowl with Sautéed Shrimp, Broccoli, and Mushrooms

Recipe 1:

Classic Baked Chicken with Herb-Roasted Potatoes

Recipe 2:

Baked Chicken with Herb-Roasted Potatoes and Carrots

Recipe 3:

Baked Chicken with Herb-Roasted Potatoes and Green Beans

Recipe 4:

Baked Chicken with Herb-Roasted Potatoes and Brussels Sprouts

Recipe 1:

Classic Baked Chicken with Herb-Roasted Potatoes

Recipe 2:

Baked Chicken with Herb-Roasted Potatoes and Carrots

Recipe 3:

Baked Chicken with Herb-Roasted Potatoes and Green Beans

Recipe 4:

Baked Chicken with Herb-Roasted Potatoes and Brussels Sprouts

Recipe 1:

Classic Grilled Pork Chops with Steamed Asparagus

Grilled Pork Chops with Steamed Asparagus and Cherry Tomatoes

Recipe 3:

Grilled Pork Chops with Steamed Asparagus and Parmesan

Recipe 4:

Grilled Pork Chops with Steamed Asparagus and Lemon Zest

CHAPTER ONE

Breakfast Recipes

Oatmeal with Berries and Nuts

Recipe 1:

Classic Oatmeal with Mixed Berries and Almonds

Ingredients:

- 1 cup rolled oats
- 2 cups water or milk (your choice)
- 1/2 cup mixed berries (strawberries, blueberries, raspberries)
- 1/4 cup sliced almonds
- 1 tablespoon honey or maple syrup (optional)
- Pinch of salt

Instructions:

1. In a medium saucepan, bring water or milk to a boil.

2. Stir in the oats and salt, reduce heat to medium-low, and cook for 5 minutes, stirring occasionally.
3. Remove from heat, cover, and let sit for 2-3 minutes.
4. Stir in the honey or maple syrup if using.
5. Serve topped with mixed berries and sliced almonds.

Nutritional Information (per serving):

- Calories: 350
- Protein: 10g
- Fat: 12g
- Carbohydrates: 52g
- Fiber: 8g
- Sugar: 14g

Cooking Time: 10 minutes
Serving Size: 2 servings

Recipe 2:

Blueberry Walnut Oatmeal

Ingredients:

- 1 cup steel-cut oats
- 3 cups water

- 1/2 cup fresh or frozen blueberries
- 1/4 cup chopped walnuts
- 1 teaspoon cinnamon
- 1 tablespoon maple syrup (optional)

Instructions:

1. In a medium saucepan, bring water to a boil.
2. Stir in the steel-cut oats, reduce heat to medium-low, and cook for 20-25 minutes, stirring occasionally.
3. Add cinnamon and cook for another 5 minutes.
4. Remove from heat and let sit for 2 minutes.
5. Stir in the maple syrup if using.
6. Serve topped with blueberries and chopped walnuts.

Nutritional Information (per serving):

- Calories: 320
- Protein: 9g
- Fat: 14g
- Carbohydrates: 43g
- Fiber: 7g
- Sugar: 10g

Cooking Time: 30 minutes
Serving Size: 2 servings

Recipe 3:

Strawberry Pecan Oatmeal

Ingredients:

- 1 cup quick oats
- 2 cups almond milk
- 1/2 cup sliced strawberries
- 1/4 cup chopped pecans
- 1 teaspoon vanilla extract
- 1 tablespoon agave syrup (optional)

Instructions:

1. In a medium saucepan, bring almond milk to a boil.
2. Stir in the quick oats and vanilla extract, reduce heat to medium-low, and cook for 1-2 minutes, stirring constantly.
3. Remove from heat and let sit for 1-2 minutes.
4. Stir in the agave syrup if using.

5. Serve topped with sliced strawberries and chopped pecans.

Nutritional Information (per serving):

- Calories: 290
- Protein: 7g
- Fat: 12g
- Carbohydrates: 39g
- Fiber: 6g
- Sugar: 12g

Cooking Time: 5 minutes
Serving Size: 2 servings

Recipe 4:

Raspberry Hazelnut Oatmeal

Ingredients:

- 1 cup old-fashioned oats
- 2 cups coconut milk
- 1/2 cup fresh raspberries
- 1/4 cup chopped hazelnuts
- 1 teaspoon chia seeds
- 1 tablespoon honey (optional)

Instructions:

1. In a medium saucepan, bring coconut milk to a boil.
2. Stir in the oats and reduce heat to medium-low, cooking for 5 minutes while stirring occasionally.
3. Add chia seeds and cook for an additional 2 minutes.
4. Remove from heat and let sit for 2-3 minutes.
5. Stir in the honey if using.
6. Serve topped with fresh raspberries and chopped hazelnuts.

Nutritional Information (per serving):

- Calories: 330
- Protein: 8g
- Fat: 15g
- Carbohydrates: 41g
- Fiber: 8g
- Sugar: 13g

Cooking Time: 10 minutes
Serving Size: 2 servings

Vegetable Frittata

Recipe 1:

Classic Vegetable Frittata

Ingredients:

- 8 large eggs
- 1/4 cup milk
- 1 cup diced bell peppers (any color)
- 1 cup chopped spinach
- 1/2 cup diced onions
- 1/2 cup cherry tomatoes, halved
- 1/2 cup shredded cheddar cheese
- 1 tablespoon olive oil
- Salt and pepper to taste

Instructions:

1. Preheat the oven to 375°F (190°C).
2. In a large bowl, whisk together the eggs, milk, salt, and pepper.
3. Heat olive oil in an oven-safe skillet over medium heat.

4. Add onions and bell peppers, cooking until softened (about 5 minutes).
5. Add spinach and cook until wilted (about 2 minutes).
6. Pour the egg mixture into the skillet and cook until the edges start to set (about 3-4 minutes).
7. Sprinkle cherry tomatoes and shredded cheddar cheese on top.
8. Transfer the skillet to the oven and bake until the frittata is fully set (about 10-12 minutes).
9. Let cool slightly before slicing and serving.

Nutritional Information (per serving):

- Calories: 200
- Protein: 14g
- Fat: 14g
- Carbohydrates: 6g
- Fiber: 2g
- Sugar: 3g

Cooking Time: 25 minutes
Serving Size: 4 servings

Recipe 2:

Broccoli and Mushroom Frittata

Ingredients:

- 8 large eggs
- 1/4 cup milk
- 1 cup chopped broccoli florets
- 1 cup sliced mushrooms
- 1/2 cup diced onions
- 1/2 cup grated Parmesan cheese
- 1 tablespoon butter
- Salt and pepper to taste

Instructions:

1. Preheat the oven to 375°F (190°C).
2. In a large bowl, whisk together the eggs, milk, salt, and pepper.
3. Heat butter in an oven-safe skillet over medium heat.
4. Add onions and cook until softened (about 3 minutes).
5. Add broccoli and mushrooms, cooking until tender (about 5 minutes).

6. Pour the egg mixture into the skillet and cook until the edges start to set (about 3-4 minutes).
7. Sprinkle grated Parmesan cheese on top.
8. Transfer the skillet to the oven and bake until the frittata is fully set (about 10-12 minutes).
9. Let cool slightly before slicing and serving.

Nutritional Information (per serving):

- Calories: 190
- Protein: 13g
- Fat: 13g
- Carbohydrates: 6g
- Fiber: 2g
- Sugar: 2g

Cooking Time: 25 minutes
Serving Size: 4 servings

Recipe 3:

Zucchini and Tomato Frittata

Ingredients:

- 8 large eggs
- 1/4 cup milk
- 1 cup sliced zucchini
- 1 cup halved cherry tomatoes
- 1/2 cup diced onions
- 1/2 cup crumbled feta cheese
- 1 tablespoon olive oil
- Salt and pepper to taste

Instructions:

1. Preheat the oven to 375°F (190°C).
2. In a large bowl, whisk together the eggs, milk, salt, and pepper.
3. Heat olive oil in an oven-safe skillet over medium heat.
4. Add onions and cook until softened (about 3 minutes).
5. Add zucchini and cook until tender (about 5 minutes).
6. Pour the egg mixture into the skillet and cook until the edges start to set (about 3-4 minutes).
7. Sprinkle cherry tomatoes and crumbled feta cheese on top.
8. Transfer the skillet to the oven and bake until the frittata is fully set (about 10-12 minutes).

9. Let cool slightly before slicing and serving.

Nutritional Information (per serving):

- Calories: 180
- Protein: 12g
- Fat: 13g
- Carbohydrates: 5g
- Fiber: 1g
- Sugar: 3g

Cooking Time: 25 minutes
Serving Size: 4 servings

Recipe 4:

Spinach and Red Pepper Frittata

Ingredients:

- 8 large eggs
- 1/4 cup milk
- 1 cup chopped spinach
- 1 cup diced red bell pepper
- 1/2 cup diced onions
- 1/2 cup shredded mozzarella cheese

- 1 tablespoon olive oil
- Salt and pepper to taste

Instructions:

1. Preheat the oven to 375°F (190°C).
2. In a large bowl, whisk together the eggs, milk, salt, and pepper.
3. Heat olive oil in an oven-safe skillet over medium heat.
4. Add onions and red bell pepper, cooking until softened (about 5 minutes).
5. Add spinach and cook until wilted (about 2 minutes).
6. Pour the egg mixture into the skillet and cook until the edges start to set (about 3-4 minutes).
7. Sprinkle shredded mozzarella cheese on top.
8. Transfer the skillet to the oven and bake until the frittata is fully set (about 10-12 minutes).
9. Let cool slightly before slicing and serving.

Nutritional Information (per serving):

- Calories: 190

- Protein: 13g
- Fat: 13g
- Carbohydrates: 5g
- Fiber: 1g
- Sugar: 3g

Cooking Time: 25 minutes
Serving Size: 4 servings

Whole Wheat Toast with Avocado and Poached Egg

Recipe 1:

Classic Whole Wheat Toast with Avocado and Poached Egg

Ingredients:

- 2 slices whole wheat bread
- 1 ripe avocado
- 2 large eggs
- 1 tablespoon white vinegar
- Salt and pepper to taste
- Red pepper flakes (optional)

Instructions:

1. Toast the whole wheat bread slices until golden brown.
2. Cut the avocado in half, remove the pit, and scoop out the flesh into a bowl. Mash with a fork and season with salt and pepper.
3. Spread the mashed avocado evenly on the toasted bread slices.
4. Fill a medium saucepan with water and bring to a gentle simmer. Add the white vinegar.
5. Crack each egg into a small bowl or cup. Create a gentle whirlpool in the water with a spoon and carefully slide each egg into the water. Poach the eggs for about 3-

4 minutes until the whites are set and the yolks are still runny.
6. Remove the poached eggs with a slotted spoon and place them on top of the avocado toast.
7. Sprinkle with red pepper flakes if desired, and serve immediately.

Nutritional Information (per serving):

- Calories: 350
- Protein: 14g
- Fat: 22g
- Carbohydrates: 29g
- Fiber: 8g
- Sugar: 2g

Cooking Time: 10 minutes
Serving Size: 2 servings

Recipe 2:

Whole Wheat Toast with Avocado, Poached Egg, and Cherry Tomatoes

Ingredients:

- 2 slices whole wheat bread
- 1 ripe avocado

- 2 large eggs
- 1 tablespoon white vinegar
- 1/2 cup halved cherry tomatoes
- 1 tablespoon olive oil
- Salt and pepper to taste
- Fresh basil leaves (optional)

Instructions:

1. Toast the whole wheat bread slices until golden brown.
2. Cut the avocado in half, remove the pit, and scoop out the flesh into a bowl. Mash with a fork and season with salt and pepper.
3. Spread the mashed avocado evenly on the toasted bread slices.
4. In a small bowl, toss the halved cherry tomatoes with olive oil, salt, and pepper.
5. Fill a medium saucepan with water and bring to a gentle simmer. Add the white vinegar.
6. Crack each egg into a small bowl or cup. Create a gentle whirlpool in the water with a spoon and carefully slide each egg into the water. Poach the eggs for about 3-

4 minutes until the whites are set and the yolks are still runny.
7. Remove the poached eggs with a slotted spoon and place them on top of the avocado toast.
8. Top with the cherry tomatoes and fresh basil leaves if desired. Serve immediately.

Nutritional Information (per serving):

- Calories: 380
- Protein: 15g
- Fat: 24g
- Carbohydrates: 31g
- Fiber: 9g
- Sugar: 3g

Cooking Time: 15 minutes
Serving Size: 2 servings

Recipe 3:

Whole Wheat Toast with Avocado, Poached Egg, and Feta Cheese

Ingredients:

- 2 slices whole wheat bread
- 1 ripe avocado

- 2 large eggs
- 1 tablespoon white vinegar
- 1/4 cup crumbled feta cheese
- Salt and pepper to taste
- Fresh dill or parsley (optional)

Instructions:

1. Toast the whole wheat bread slices until golden brown.
2. Cut the avocado in half, remove the pit, and scoop out the flesh into a bowl. Mash with a fork and season with salt and pepper.
3. Spread the mashed avocado evenly on the toasted bread slices.
4. Fill a medium saucepan with water and bring to a gentle simmer. Add the white vinegar.
5. Crack each egg into a small bowl or cup. Create a gentle whirlpool in the water with a spoon and carefully slide each egg into the water. Poach the eggs for about 3-4 minutes until the whites are set and the yolks are still runny.
6. Remove the poached eggs with a slotted spoon and place them on top of the avocado toast.

7. Sprinkle the crumbled feta cheese over the eggs and top with fresh dill or parsley if desired. Serve immediately.

Nutritional Information (per serving):

- Calories: 370
- Protein: 17g
- Fat: 25g
- Carbohydrates: 28g
- Fiber: 8g
- Sugar: 2g

Cooking Time: 10 minutes
Serving Size: 2 servings

Recipe 4:

Whole Wheat Toast with Avocado, Poached Egg, and Smoked Salmon

Ingredients:

- 2 slices whole wheat bread
- 1 ripe avocado
- 2 large eggs
- 1 tablespoon white vinegar
- 2 ounces smoked salmon
- 1 teaspoon capers (optional)

- Salt and pepper to taste
- Lemon wedges for serving

Instructions:

1. Toast the whole wheat bread slices until golden brown.
2. Cut the avocado in half, remove the pit, and scoop out the flesh into a bowl. Mash with a fork and season with salt and pepper.
3. Spread the mashed avocado evenly on the toasted bread slices.
4. Fill a medium saucepan with water and bring to a gentle simmer. Add the white vinegar.
5. Crack each egg into a small bowl or cup. Create a gentle whirlpool in the water with a spoon and carefully slide each egg into the water. Poach the eggs for about 3-4 minutes until the whites are set and the yolks are still runny.
6. Remove the poached eggs with a slotted spoon and place them on top of the avocado toast.
7. Layer the smoked salmon over the poached eggs and sprinkle with capers if desired.

8. Serve with lemon wedges and enjoy immediately.

Nutritional Information (per serving):

- Calories: 390
- Protein: 19g
- Fat: 26g
- Carbohydrates: 29g
- Fiber: 8g
- Sugar: 2g

Cooking Time: 10 minutes
Serving Size: 2 servings

Greek Yogurt with Granola and Kiwi

Recipe 1: Classic Greek Yogurt with Granola and Kiwi

Ingredients:

- 1 cup plain Greek yogurt
- 1/2 cup granola
- 2 kiwis, peeled and sliced
- 1 tablespoon honey (optional)

Instructions:

1. Spoon the Greek yogurt into a bowl.
2. Top with granola and sliced kiwis.
3. Drizzle with honey if desired.
4. Serve immediately.

Nutritional Information (per serving):

- Calories: 300
- Protein: 15g
- Fat: 10g
- Carbohydrates: 40g
- Fiber: 5g
- Sugar: 20g

Cooking Time: 5 minutes
Serving Size: 1 serving

Recipe 2:

Greek Yogurt with Granola, Kiwi, and Berries

Ingredients:

- 1 cup plain Greek yogurt
- 1/2 cup granola
- 2 kiwis, peeled and sliced
- 1/2 cup mixed berries (strawberries, blueberries, raspberries)
- 1 tablespoon maple syrup (optional)

Instructions:

1. Spoon the Greek yogurt into a bowl.
2. Top with granola, sliced kiwis, and mixed berries.
3. Drizzle with maple syrup if desired.
4. Serve immediately.

Nutritional Information (per serving):

- Calories: 330
- Protein: 16g

- Fat: 11g
- Carbohydrates: 45g
- Fiber: 7g
- Sugar: 22g

Cooking Time: 5 minutes
Serving Size: 1 serving

Recipe 3:

Greek Yogurt with Granola, Kiwi, and Almonds

Ingredients:

- 1 cup plain Greek yogurt
- 1/2 cup granola
- 2 kiwis, peeled and sliced
- 1/4 cup sliced almonds
- 1 teaspoon chia seeds
- 1 tablespoon agave syrup (optional)

Instructions:

1. Spoon the Greek yogurt into a bowl.
2. Top with granola, sliced kiwis, sliced almonds, and chia seeds.

3. Drizzle with agave syrup if desired.
4. Serve immediately.

Nutritional Information (per serving):

- Calories: 340
- Protein: 17g
- Fat: 14g
- Carbohydrates: 40g
- Fiber: 8g
- Sugar: 19g

Cooking Time: 5 minutes
Serving Size: 1 serving

Recipe 4:

Greek Yogurt with Granola, Kiwi, and Coconut

Ingredients:

- 1 cup plain Greek yogurt
- 1/2 cup granola
- 2 kiwis, peeled and sliced
- 1/4 cup shredded coconut
- 1 tablespoon honey (optional)

Instructions:

1. Spoon the Greek yogurt into a bowl.
2. Top with granola, sliced kiwis, and shredded coconut.
3. Drizzle with honey if desired.
4. Serve immediately.

Nutritional Information (per serving):

- Calories: 350
- Protein: 16g
- Fat: 15g
- Carbohydrates: 40g
- Fiber: 7g
- Sugar: 21g

Cooking Time: 5 minutes
Serving Size: 1 serving

CHAPTER TWO

Lunch Recipes

Grilled Salmon with Roasted Vegetables

Recipe 1:

Classic Grilled Salmon with Roasted Vegetables

Ingredients:

- 2 salmon filets (6 oz each)
- 1 tablespoon olive oil
- 1 lemon, sliced
- 1 teaspoon garlic powder
- Salt and pepper to taste
- 2 cups mixed vegetables (carrots, bell peppers, zucchini)
- 1 tablespoon olive oil (for vegetables)
- 1 teaspoon dried thyme

Instructions:

1. Preheat the oven to 400°F (200°C).
2. Toss the mixed vegetables with 1 tablespoon of olive oil, dried thyme, salt, and pepper. Spread them out on a baking sheet.
3. Roast the vegetables in the preheated oven for 20-25 minutes, or until tender and slightly browned.
4. Meanwhile, preheat the grill to medium-high heat.
5. Brush the salmon filets with olive oil and season with garlic powder, salt, and pepper. Place lemon slices on top of each filet.
6. Grill the salmon for about 4-5 minutes on each side, or until the salmon is cooked through and flakes easily with a fork.
7. Serve the grilled salmon with the roasted vegetables.

Nutritional Information (per serving):

- Calories: 450
- Protein: 35g

- Fat: 25g
- Carbohydrates: 20g
- Fiber: 6g
- Sugar: 8g

Cooking Time: 30 minutes
Serving Size: 2 servings

Recipe 2:

Grilled Salmon with Roasted Brussels Sprouts and Sweet Potatoes

Ingredients:

- 2 salmon filets (6 oz each)
- 1 tablespoon olive oil
- 1 lemon, sliced
- 1 teaspoon smoked paprika
- Salt and pepper to taste
- 1 cup Brussels sprouts, halved
- 1 cup sweet potatoes, diced
- 1 tablespoon olive oil (for vegetables)
- 1 teaspoon rosemary

Instructions:

1. Preheat the oven to 400°F (200°C).

2. Toss the Brussels sprouts and sweet potatoes with 1 tablespoon of olive oil, rosemary, salt, and pepper. Spread them out on a baking sheet.
3. Roast the vegetables in the preheated oven for 25-30 minutes, or until tender and slightly browned.
4. Meanwhile, preheat the grill to medium-high heat.
5. Brush the salmon filets with olive oil and season with smoked paprika, salt, and pepper. Place lemon slices on top of each filet.
6. Grill the salmon for about 4-5 minutes on each side, or until the salmon is cooked through and flakes easily with a fork.
7. Serve the grilled salmon with the roasted Brussels sprouts and sweet potatoes.

Nutritional Information (per serving):

- Calories: 480
- Protein: 36g
- Fat: 26g
- Carbohydrates: 28g

- Fiber: 7g
- Sugar: 9g

Cooking Time: 35 minutes
Serving Size: 2 servings

Recipe 3:

Grilled Salmon with Roasted Asparagus and Cherry Tomatoes

Ingredients:

- 2 salmon filets (6 oz each)
- 1 tablespoon olive oil
- 1 lemon, sliced
- 1 teaspoon dill
- Salt and pepper to taste
- 1 bunch asparagus, trimmed
- 1 cup cherry tomatoes, halved
- 1 tablespoon olive oil (for vegetables)
- 1 teaspoon balsamic vinegar

Instructions:

1. Preheat the oven to 400°F (200°C).

2. Toss the asparagus and cherry tomatoes with 1 tablespoon of olive oil, balsamic vinegar, salt, and pepper. Spread them out on a baking sheet.
3. Roast the vegetables in the preheated oven for 15-20 minutes, or until tender and slightly browned.
4. Meanwhile, preheat the grill to medium-high heat.
5. Brush the salmon filets with olive oil and season with dill, salt, and pepper. Place lemon slices on top of each filet.
6. Grill the salmon for about 4-5 minutes on each side, or until the salmon is cooked through and flakes easily with a fork.
7. Serve the grilled salmon with the roasted asparagus and cherry tomatoes.

Nutritional Information (per serving):

- Calories: 430
- Protein: 34g
- Fat: 24g
- Carbohydrates: 16g

- Fiber: 5g
- Sugar: 7g

Cooking Time: 25 minutes
Serving Size: 2 servings

Recipe 4:

Grilled Salmon with Roasted Broccoli and Red Bell Peppers

Ingredients:

- 2 salmon filets (6 oz each)
- 1 tablespoon olive oil
- 1 lemon, sliced
- 1 teaspoon cumin
- Salt and pepper to taste
- 1 cup broccoli florets
- 1 cup red bell peppers, sliced
- 1 tablespoon olive oil (for vegetables)
- 1 teaspoon oregano

Instructions:

1. Preheat the oven to 400°F (200°C).

2. Toss the broccoli florets and red bell peppers with 1 tablespoon of olive oil, oregano, salt, and pepper. Spread them out on a baking sheet.
3. Roast the vegetables in the preheated oven for 20-25 minutes, or until tender and slightly browned.
4. Meanwhile, preheat the grill to medium-high heat.
5. Brush the salmon filets with olive oil and season with cumin, salt, and pepper. Place lemon slices on top of each filet.
6. Grill the salmon for about 4-5 minutes on each side, or until the salmon is cooked through and flakes easily with a fork.
7. Serve the grilled salmon with the roasted broccoli and red bell peppers.

Nutritional Information (per serving):

- Calories: 440
- Protein: 35g
- Fat: 25g
- Carbohydrates: 18g

- Fiber: 6g
- Sugar: 6g

Cooking Time: 30 minutes
Serving Size: 2 servings

Quinoa and Spinach Salad with Feta

Recipe 1:

Classic Quinoa and Spinach Salad with Feta

Ingredients:

- 1 cup quinoa, rinsed
- 2 cups water
- 4 cups fresh spinach, chopped
- 1/2 cup crumbled feta cheese
- 1/4 cup red onion, finely chopped
- 1/4 cup olive oil
- 2 tablespoons lemon juice
- 1 clove garlic, minced
- Salt and pepper to taste

Instructions:

1. In a medium saucepan, bring the quinoa and water to a boil. Reduce heat, cover, and simmer for about 15 minutes, or until the water is absorbed and the quinoa is tender.
2. Let the quinoa cool to room temperature.
3. In a large bowl, combine the cooked quinoa, chopped spinach, crumbled feta cheese, and red onion.
4. In a small bowl, whisk together the olive oil, lemon juice, minced garlic, salt, and pepper.
5. Pour the dressing over the salad and toss to combine.
6. Serve immediately or refrigerate until ready to serve.

Nutritional Information (per serving):

- Calories: 320
- Protein: 9g
- Fat: 19g
- Carbohydrates: 30g
- Fiber: 4g

- Sugar: 2g

Cooking Time: 25 minutes
Serving Size: 4 servings

Recipe 2:

Quinoa and Spinach Salad with Feta and Cherry Tomatoes

Ingredients:

- 1 cup quinoa, rinsed
- 2 cups water
- 4 cups fresh spinach, chopped
- 1/2 cup crumbled feta cheese
- 1 cup cherry tomatoes, halved
- 1/4 cup red onion, finely chopped
- 1/4 cup olive oil
- 2 tablespoons balsamic vinegar
- Salt and pepper to taste

Instructions:

1. In a medium saucepan, bring the quinoa and water to a boil. Reduce heat, cover, and simmer for about 15 minutes, or until the

water is absorbed and the quinoa is tender.
2. Let the quinoa cool to room temperature.
3. In a large bowl, combine the cooked quinoa, chopped spinach, crumbled feta cheese, cherry tomatoes, and red onion.
4. In a small bowl, whisk together the olive oil, balsamic vinegar, salt, and pepper.
5. Pour the dressing over the salad and toss to combine.
6. Serve immediately or refrigerate until ready to serve.

Nutritional Information (per serving):

- Calories: 330
- Protein: 10g
- Fat: 19g
- Carbohydrates: 31g
- Fiber: 4g
- Sugar: 3g

Cooking Time: 25 minutes
Serving Size: 4 servings

Recipe 3:

Quinoa and Spinach Salad with Feta and Avocado

Ingredients:

- 1 cup quinoa, rinsed
- 2 cups water
- 4 cups fresh spinach, chopped
- 1/2 cup crumbled feta cheese
- 1 ripe avocado, diced
- 1/4 cup red onion, finely chopped
- 1/4 cup olive oil
- 2 tablespoons lime juice
- 1 clove garlic, minced
- Salt and pepper to taste

Instructions:

1. In a medium saucepan, bring the quinoa and water to a boil. Reduce heat, cover, and simmer for about 15 minutes, or until the water is absorbed and the quinoa is tender.
2. Let the quinoa cool to room temperature.
3. In a large bowl, combine the cooked quinoa, chopped spinach, crumbled feta cheese, diced avocado, and red onion.

4. In a small bowl, whisk together the olive oil, lime juice, minced garlic, salt, and pepper.
5. Pour the dressing over the salad and toss to combine.
6. Serve immediately or refrigerate until ready to serve.

Nutritional Information (per serving):

- Calories: 350
- Protein: 10g
- Fat: 23g
- Carbohydrates: 29g
- Fiber: 7g
- Sugar: 2g

Cooking Time: 25 minutes
Serving Size: 4 servings

Recipe 4:

Quinoa and Spinach Salad with Feta and Cucumbers

Ingredients:

- 1 cup quinoa, rinsed
- 2 cups water
- 4 cups fresh spinach, chopped

- 1/2 cup crumbled feta cheese
- 1 cup cucumber, diced
- 1/4 cup red onion, finely chopped
- 1/4 cup olive oil
- 2 tablespoons red wine vinegar
- 1 teaspoon dried oregano
- Salt and pepper to taste

Instructions:

1. In a medium saucepan, bring the quinoa and water to a boil. Reduce heat, cover, and simmer for about 15 minutes, or until the water is absorbed and the quinoa is tender.
2. Let the quinoa cool to room temperature.
3. In a large bowl, combine the cooked quinoa, chopped spinach, crumbled feta cheese, diced cucumber, and red onion.
4. In a small bowl, whisk together the olive oil, red wine vinegar, dried oregano, salt, and pepper.
5. Pour the dressing over the salad and toss to combine.
6. Serve immediately or refrigerate until ready to serve.

Nutritional Information (per serving):

- Calories: 310
- Protein: 9g
- Fat: 19g
- Carbohydrates: 28g
- Fiber: 4g
- Sugar: 2g

Cooking Time: 25 minutes
Serving Size: 4 servings

Lentil and Sweet Potato Soup

Recipe 1:

Classic Lentil and Sweet Potato Soup

Ingredients:

- 1 cup lentils, rinsed
- 2 medium sweet potatoes, peeled and diced
- 1 onion, chopped
- 2 cloves garlic, minced
- 1 tablespoon olive oil
- 6 cups vegetable broth
- 1 teaspoon cumin
- 1 teaspoon paprika
- Salt and pepper to taste

Instructions:

1. In a large pot, heat the olive oil over medium heat. Add the chopped onion and minced garlic, and sauté until softened, about 5 minutes.
2. Add the diced sweet potatoes and cook for another 5 minutes.
3. Stir in the lentils, cumin, and paprika. Pour in the vegetable broth.
4. Bring the mixture to a boil, then reduce the heat and simmer for about 30 minutes, or until the

lentils and sweet potatoes are tender.
5. Season with salt and pepper to taste.
6. Serve hot.

Nutritional Information (per serving):

- Calories: 250
- Protein: 10g
- Fat: 4g
- Carbohydrates: 45g
- Fiber: 12g
- Sugar: 8g

Cooking Time: 45 minutes
Serving Size: 4 servings

Recipe 2:

Lentil and Sweet Potato Soup with Spinach

Ingredients:

- 1 cup lentils, rinsed
- 2 medium sweet potatoes, peeled and diced
- 1 onion, chopped
- 2 cloves garlic, minced
- 1 tablespoon olive oil
- 6 cups vegetable broth
- 1 teaspoon cumin
- 1 teaspoon paprika
- 4 cups fresh spinach, chopped
- Salt and pepper to taste

Instructions:

1. In a large pot, heat the olive oil over medium heat. Add the chopped onion and minced garlic, and sauté until softened, about 5 minutes.
2. Add the diced sweet potatoes and cook for another 5 minutes.
3. Stir in the lentils, cumin, and paprika. Pour in the vegetable broth.
4. Bring the mixture to a boil, then reduce the heat and simmer for about 30 minutes, or until the

lentils and sweet potatoes are tender.
5. Stir in the chopped spinach and cook for another 5 minutes.
6. Season with salt and pepper to taste.
7. Serve hot.

Nutritional Information (per serving):

- Calories: 270
- Protein: 12g
- Fat: 4g
- Carbohydrates: 48g
- Fiber: 13g
- Sugar: 8g

Cooking Time: 50 minutes
Serving Size: 4 servings

Recipe 3:

Lentil and Sweet Potato Soup with Coconut Milk

Ingredients:

- 1 cup lentils, rinsed
- 2 medium sweet potatoes, peeled and diced
- 1 onion, chopped
- 2 cloves garlic, minced
- 1 tablespoon olive oil
- 6 cups vegetable broth
- 1 teaspoon cumin
- 1 teaspoon turmeric
- 1 can (14 oz) coconut milk
- Salt and pepper to taste

Instructions:

1. In a large pot, heat the olive oil over medium heat. Add the chopped onion and minced garlic, and sauté until softened, about 5 minutes.
2. Add the diced sweet potatoes and cook for another 5 minutes.
3. Stir in the lentils, cumin, and turmeric. Pour in the vegetable broth.
4. Bring the mixture to a boil, then reduce the heat and simmer for about 30 minutes, or until the lentils and sweet potatoes are tender.

5. Stir in the coconut milk and cook for another 5 minutes.
6. Season with salt and pepper to taste.
7. Serve hot.

Nutritional Information (per serving):

- Calories: 320
- Protein: 12g
- Fat: 12g
- Carbohydrates: 45g
- Fiber: 12g
- Sugar: 8g

Cooking Time: 50 minutes
Serving Size: 4 servings

Recipe 4:

Spicy Lentil and Sweet Potato Soup

Ingredients:

- 1 cup lentils, rinsed
- 2 medium sweet potatoes, peeled and diced
- 1 onion, chopped
- 2 cloves garlic, minced
- 1 tablespoon olive oil

- 6 cups vegetable broth
- 1 teaspoon cumin
- 1 teaspoon smoked paprika
- 1/2 teaspoon cayenne pepper (optional, for heat)
- 1 can (14 oz) diced tomatoes
- Salt and pepper to taste

Instructions:

1. In a large pot, heat the olive oil over medium heat. Add the chopped onion and minced garlic, and sauté until softened, about 5 minutes.
2. Add the diced sweet potatoes and cook for another 5 minutes.
3. Stir in the lentils, cumin, smoked paprika, and cayenne pepper. Pour in the vegetable broth and add the diced tomatoes.
4. Bring the mixture to a boil, then reduce the heat and simmer for about 30 minutes, or until the lentils and sweet potatoes are tender.
5. Season with salt and pepper to taste.
6. Serve hot.

Nutritional Information (per serving):

- Calories: 270
- Protein: 11g
- Fat: 4g
- Carbohydrates: 46g
- Fiber: 12g
- Sugar: 9g

Cooking Time: 45 minutes
Serving Size: 4 servings

Brown Rice Bowl with Sautéed Shrimp and Broccoli

Recipe 1: Classic Brown Rice Bowl with Sautéed Shrimp and Broccoli

Ingredients:

- 1 cup brown rice
- 2 cups water
- 1 pound shrimp, peeled and deveined
- 2 cups broccoli florets
- 2 tablespoons olive oil
- 2 cloves garlic, minced
- 1 tablespoon soy sauce
- 1 tablespoon lemon juice
- Salt and pepper to taste

Instructions:

1. In a medium saucepan, bring the brown rice and water to a boil. Reduce heat, cover, and simmer for about 40-45 minutes, or until the water is absorbed and the rice is tender.
2. While the rice is cooking, heat 1 tablespoon of olive oil in a large skillet over medium heat. Add the broccoli florets and sauté for about 5-7 minutes, or until tender. Remove from the skillet and set aside.

3. In the same skillet, heat the remaining tablespoon of olive oil. Add the minced garlic and sauté for about 1 minute.
4. Add the shrimp to the skillet and cook for about 3-4 minutes on each side, or until the shrimp is pink and opaque.
5. Stir in the soy sauce and lemon juice. Season with salt and pepper to taste.
6. Serve the sautéed shrimp and broccoli over the cooked brown rice.

Nutritional Information (per serving):

- Calories: 400
- Protein: 30g
- Fat: 14g
- Carbohydrates: 41g
- Fiber: 4g
- Sugar: 1g

Cooking Time: 50 minutes
Serving Size: 4 servings

Recipe 2:

Brown Rice Bowl with Sautéed Shrimp, Broccoli, and Carrots

Ingredients:

- 1 cup brown rice
- 2 cups water
- 1 pound shrimp, peeled and deveined
- 2 cups broccoli florets
- 1 cup carrots, sliced
- 2 tablespoons olive oil
- 2 cloves garlic, minced
- 1 tablespoon soy sauce
- 1 tablespoon sesame oil
- Salt and pepper to taste

Instructions:

1. In a medium saucepan, bring the brown rice and water to a boil. Reduce heat, cover, and simmer for about 40-45 minutes, or until the water is absorbed and the rice is tender.
2. While the rice is cooking, heat 1 tablespoon of olive oil in a large skillet over medium heat. Add the broccoli florets and carrots, and sauté for about 5-7 minutes, or

until tender. Remove from the skillet and set aside.
3. In the same skillet, heat the remaining tablespoon of olive oil. Add the minced garlic and sauté for about 1 minute.
4. Add the shrimp to the skillet and cook for about 3-4 minutes on each side, or until the shrimp is pink and opaque.
5. Stir in the soy sauce and sesame oil. Season with salt and pepper to taste.
6. Serve the sautéed shrimp, broccoli, and carrots over the cooked brown rice.

Nutritional Information (per serving):

- Calories: 420
- Protein: 30g
- Fat: 15g
- Carbohydrates: 43g
- Fiber: 5g
- Sugar: 3g

Cooking Time: 50 minutes
Serving Size: 4 servings

Recipe 3:

Brown Rice Bowl with Sautéed Shrimp, Broccoli, and Bell Peppers

Ingredients:

- 1 cup brown rice
- 2 cups water
- 1 pound shrimp, peeled and deveined
- 2 cups broccoli florets
- 1 cup bell peppers, sliced
- 2 tablespoons olive oil
- 2 cloves garlic, minced
- 1 tablespoon soy sauce
- 1 tablespoon rice vinegar
- Salt and pepper to taste

Instructions:

1. In a medium saucepan, bring the brown rice and water to a boil. Reduce heat, cover, and simmer for about 40-45 minutes, or until the water is absorbed and the rice is tender.
2. While the rice is cooking, heat 1 tablespoon of olive oil in a large skillet over medium heat. Add the

broccoli florets and bell peppers, and sauté for about 5-7 minutes, or until tender. Remove from the skillet and set aside.
3. In the same skillet, heat the remaining tablespoon of olive oil. Add the minced garlic and sauté for about 1 minute.
4. Add the shrimp to the skillet and cook for about 3-4 minutes on each side, or until the shrimp is pink and opaque.
5. Stir in the soy sauce and rice vinegar. Season with salt and pepper to taste.
6. Serve the sautéed shrimp, broccoli, and bell peppers over the cooked brown rice.

Nutritional Information (per serving):

- Calories: 410
- Protein: 30g
- Fat: 14g
- Carbohydrates: 42g
- Fiber: 4g
- Sugar: 2g

Cooking Time: 50 minutes
Serving Size: 4 servings

Recipe 4:

Brown Rice Bowl with Sautéed Shrimp, Broccoli, and Mushrooms

Ingredients:

- 1 cup brown rice
- 2 cups water
- 1 pound shrimp, peeled and deveined
- 2 cups broccoli florets
- 1 cup mushrooms, sliced
- 2 tablespoons olive oil
- 2 cloves garlic, minced
- 1 tablespoon soy sauce
- 1 tablespoon lime juice
- Salt and pepper to taste

Instructions:

1. In a medium saucepan, bring the brown rice and water to a boil. Reduce heat, cover, and simmer for about 40-45 minutes, or until the water is absorbed and the rice is tender.
2. While the rice is cooking, heat 1 tablespoon of olive oil in a large skillet over medium heat. Add the broccoli florets and mushrooms, and sauté for about 5-7 minutes, or until tender. Remove from the skillet and set aside.
3. In the same skillet, heat the remaining tablespoon of olive oil. Add the minced garlic and sauté for about 1 minute.
4. Add the shrimp to the skillet and cook for about 3-4 minutes on each side, or until the shrimp is pink and opaque.
5. Stir in the soy sauce and lime juice. Season with salt and pepper to taste.
6. Serve the sautéed shrimp, broccoli, and mushrooms over the cooked brown rice.

Nutritional Information (per serving):

- Calories: 400
- Protein: 30g
- Fat: 14g
- Carbohydrates: 41g
- Fiber: 4g
- Sugar: 2g

Cooking Time: 50 minutes
Serving Size: 4 servings

CHAPTER THREE

Dinner Recipes

Baked Chicken with Herb-Roasted Potatoes

Recipe 1:

Classic Baked Chicken with Herb-Roasted Potatoes

Ingredients:

- 4 chicken breasts
- 2 pounds potatoes, diced
- 2 tablespoons olive oil
- 2 teaspoons dried rosemary
- 2 teaspoons dried thyme
- 2 cloves garlic, minced
- Salt and pepper to taste

Instructions:

1. Preheat the oven to 400°F (200°C).
2. In a large bowl, combine the diced potatoes, olive oil, rosemary, thyme, minced garlic, salt, and pepper. Toss to coat.
3. Spread the potatoes in a single layer on a baking sheet.
4. Place the chicken breasts on another baking sheet and season with salt and pepper.
5. Bake the potatoes and chicken in the preheated oven for about 30-35 minutes, or until the chicken is cooked through and the potatoes are golden and crispy.
6. Serve the baked chicken with the herb-roasted potatoes.

Nutritional Information (per serving):

- Calories: 420
- Protein: 35g
- Fat: 12g
- Carbohydrates: 45g
- Fiber: 5g
- Sugar: 2g

Cooking Time: 45 minutes
Serving Size: 4 servings

Recipe 2:

Baked Chicken with Herb-Roasted Potatoes and Carrots

Ingredients:

- 4 chicken breasts
- 2 pounds potatoes, diced
- 1 pound carrots, sliced
- 2 tablespoons olive oil
- 2 teaspoons dried rosemary
- 2 teaspoons dried thyme
- 2 cloves garlic, minced
- Salt and pepper to taste

Instructions:

1. Preheat the oven to 400°F (200°C).
2. In a large bowl, combine the diced potatoes, sliced carrots, olive oil, rosemary, thyme, minced garlic, salt, and pepper. Toss to coat.
3. Spread the potatoes and carrots in a single layer on a baking sheet.

4. Place the chicken breasts on another baking sheet and season with salt and pepper.
5. Bake the potatoes, carrots, and chicken in the preheated oven for about 30-35 minutes, or until the chicken is cooked through and the vegetables are golden and crispy.
6. Serve the baked chicken with the herb-roasted potatoes and carrots.

Nutritional Information (per serving):

- Calories: 450
- Protein: 35g
- Fat: 12g
- Carbohydrates: 50g
- Fiber: 6g
- Sugar: 5g

Cooking Time: 45 minutes
Serving Size: 4 servings

Recipe 3:

Baked Chicken with Herb-Roasted Potatoes and Green Beans

Ingredients:

- 4 chicken breasts
- 2 pounds potatoes, diced
- 1 pound green beans, trimmed
- 2 tablespoons olive oil
- 2 teaspoons dried rosemary
- 2 teaspoons dried thyme
- 2 cloves garlic, minced
- Salt and pepper to taste

Instructions:

1. Preheat the oven to 400°F (200°C).
2. In a large bowl, combine the diced potatoes, olive oil, rosemary, thyme, minced garlic, salt, and pepper. Toss to coat.
3. Spread the potatoes in a single layer on a baking sheet.
4. Place the chicken breasts on another baking sheet and season with salt and pepper.
5. Bake the potatoes and chicken in the preheated oven for about 25 minutes.
6. Add the green beans to the baking sheet with the potatoes, tossing them lightly with the oil and herbs.

7. Continue baking for another 10-15 minutes, or until the chicken is cooked through and the vegetables are tender.
8. Serve the baked chicken with the herb-roasted potatoes and green beans.

Nutritional Information (per serving):

- Calories: 430
- Protein: 35g
- Fat: 12g
- Carbohydrates: 46g
- Fiber: 7g
- Sugar: 3g

Cooking Time: 45 minutes
Serving Size: 4 servings

Recipe 4:

Baked Chicken with Herb-Roasted Potatoes and Brussels Sprouts

Ingredients:

- 4 chicken breasts

- 2 pounds potatoes, diced
- 1 pound Brussels sprouts, halved
- 2 tablespoons olive oil
- 2 teaspoons dried rosemary
- 2 teaspoons dried thyme
- 2 cloves garlic, minced
- Salt and pepper to taste

Instructions:

1. Preheat the oven to 400°F (200°C).
2. In a large bowl, combine the diced potatoes, halved Brussels sprouts, olive oil, rosemary, thyme, minced garlic, salt, and pepper. Toss to coat.
3. Spread the potatoes and Brussels sprouts in a single layer on a baking sheet.
4. Place the chicken breasts on another baking sheet and season with salt and pepper.
5. Bake the potatoes, Brussels sprouts, and chicken in the preheated oven for about 30-35 minutes, or until the chicken is cooked through and the vegetables are golden and crispy.

6. Serve the baked chicken with the herb-roasted potatoes and Brussels sprouts.

Nutritional Information (per serving):

- Calories: 440
- Protein: 35g
- Fat: 13g
- Carbohydrates: 47g
- Fiber: 8g
- Sugar: 3g

Cooking Time: 45 minutes
Serving Size: 4 servings

Spaghetti Squash with Marinara and Turkey Meatballs

Recipe 1:

Classic Baked Chicken with Herb-Roasted Potatoes

Ingredients:

- 4 chicken breasts
- 2 pounds potatoes, diced
- 2 tablespoons olive oil
- 2 teaspoons dried rosemary
- 2 teaspoons dried thyme
- 2 cloves garlic, minced
- Salt and pepper to taste

Instructions:

1. Preheat the oven to 400°F (200°C).
2. In a large bowl, combine the diced potatoes, olive oil, rosemary, thyme, minced garlic, salt, and pepper. Toss to coat.
3. Spread the potatoes in a single layer on a baking sheet.
4. Place the chicken breasts on another baking sheet and season with salt and pepper.
5. Bake the potatoes and chicken in the preheated oven for about 30-

35 minutes, or until the chicken is cooked through and the potatoes are golden and crispy.
6. Serve the baked chicken with the herb-roasted potatoes.

Nutritional Information (per serving):

- Calories: 420
- Protein: 35g
- Fat: 12g
- Carbohydrates: 45g
- Fiber: 5g
- Sugar: 2g

Cooking Time: 45 minutes
Serving Size: 4 servings

Recipe 2:

Baked Chicken with Herb-Roasted Potatoes and Carrots

Ingredients:

- 4 chicken breasts
- 2 pounds potatoes, diced
- 1 pound carrots, sliced
- 2 tablespoons olive oil
- 2 teaspoons dried rosemary

- 2 teaspoons dried thyme
- 2 cloves garlic, minced
- Salt and pepper to taste

Instructions:

1. Preheat the oven to 400°F (200°C).
2. In a large bowl, combine the diced potatoes, sliced carrots, olive oil, rosemary, thyme, minced garlic, salt, and pepper. Toss to coat.
3. Spread the potatoes and carrots in a single layer on a baking sheet.
4. Place the chicken breasts on another baking sheet and season with salt and pepper.
5. Bake the potatoes, carrots, and chicken in the preheated oven for about 30-35 minutes, or until the chicken is cooked through and the vegetables are golden and crispy.
6. Serve the baked chicken with the herb-roasted potatoes and carrots.

Nutritional Information (per serving):

- Calories: 450
- Protein: 35g
- Fat: 12g

- Carbohydrates: 50g
- Fiber: 6g
- Sugar: 5g

Cooking Time: 45 minutes
Serving Size: 4 servings

Recipe 3:

Baked Chicken with Herb-Roasted Potatoes and Green Beans

Ingredients:

- 4 chicken breasts
- 2 pounds potatoes, diced
- 1 pound green beans, trimmed
- 2 tablespoons olive oil
- 2 teaspoons dried rosemary
- 2 teaspoons dried thyme
- 2 cloves garlic, minced
- Salt and pepper to taste

Instructions:

1. Preheat the oven to 400°F (200°C).
2. In a large bowl, combine the diced potatoes, olive oil, rosemary,

thyme, minced garlic, salt, and pepper. Toss to coat.
3. Spread the potatoes in a single layer on a baking sheet.
4. Place the chicken breasts on another baking sheet and season with salt and pepper.
5. Bake the potatoes and chicken in the preheated oven for about 25 minutes.
6. Add the green beans to the baking sheet with the potatoes, tossing them lightly with the oil and herbs.
7. Continue baking for another 10-15 minutes, or until the chicken is cooked through and the vegetables are tender.
8. Serve the baked chicken with the herb-roasted potatoes and green beans.

Nutritional Information (per serving):

- Calories: 430
- Protein: 35g
- Fat: 12g
- Carbohydrates: 46g
- Fiber: 7g
- Sugar: 3g

Cooking Time: 45 minutes
Serving Size: 4 servings

Recipe 4:

Baked Chicken with Herb-Roasted Potatoes and Brussels Sprouts

Ingredients:

- 4 chicken breasts
- 2 pounds potatoes, diced
- 1 pound Brussels sprouts, halved
- 2 tablespoons olive oil
- 2 teaspoons dried rosemary
- 2 teaspoons dried thyme
- 2 cloves garlic, minced
- Salt and pepper to taste

Instructions:

1. Preheat the oven to 400°F (200°C).
2. In a large bowl, combine the diced potatoes, halved Brussels sprouts, olive oil, rosemary, thyme, minced garlic, salt, and pepper. Toss to coat.
3. Spread the potatoes and Brussels sprouts in a single layer on a baking sheet.
4. Place the chicken breasts on another baking sheet and season with salt and pepper.

5. Bake the potatoes, Brussels sprouts, and chicken in the preheated oven for about 30-35 minutes, or until the chicken is cooked through and the vegetables are golden and crispy.
6. Serve the baked chicken with the herb-roasted potatoes and Brussels sprouts.

Nutritional Information (per serving):

- Calories: 440
- Protein: 35g
- Fat: 13g
- Carbohydrates: 47g
- Fiber: 8g
- Sugar: 3g

Cooking Time: 45 minutes
Serving Size: 4 serving

Grilled Pork Chops with Steamed Asparagus

Recipe 1:

Classic Grilled Pork Chops with Steamed Asparagus

Ingredients:

- 4 pork chops
- 1 pound asparagus, trimmed
- 2 tablespoons olive oil
- 2 cloves garlic, minced
- 1 tablespoon lemon juice
- Salt and pepper to taste

Instructions:

1. Preheat the grill to medium-high heat.
2. Rub the pork chops with 1 tablespoon of olive oil, minced garlic, salt, and pepper.
3. Grill the pork chops for about 5-7 minutes per side, or until the internal temperature reaches 145°F (63°C).
4. While the pork chops are grilling, steam the asparagus in a steamer basket over boiling water for about 5-7 minutes, or until tender.
5. Drizzle the steamed asparagus with the remaining tablespoon of

olive oil and lemon juice. Season with salt and pepper to taste.
6. Serve the grilled pork chops with the steamed asparagus.

Nutritional Information (per serving):

- Calories: 350
- Protein: 30g
- Fat: 20g
- Carbohydrates: 8g
- Fiber: 3g
- Sugar: 3g

Cooking Time: 25 minutes
Serving Size: 4 servings

Recipe 2:

Grilled Pork Chops with Steamed Asparagus and Cherry Tomatoes

Ingredients:

- 4 pork chops
- 1 pound asparagus, trimmed
- 1 cup cherry tomatoes, halved
- 2 tablespoons olive oil
- 2 cloves garlic, minced
- 1 tablespoon balsamic vinegar

- Salt and pepper to taste

Instructions:

1. Preheat the grill to medium-high heat.
2. Rub the pork chops with 1 tablespoon of olive oil, minced garlic, salt, and pepper.
3. Grill the pork chops for about 5-7 minutes per side, or until the internal temperature reaches 145°F (63°C).
4. While the pork chops are grilling, steam the asparagus in a steamer basket over boiling water for about 5-7 minutes, or until tender.
5. In a small bowl, toss the cherry tomatoes with the remaining tablespoon of olive oil, balsamic vinegar, salt, and pepper.
6. Serve the grilled pork chops with the steamed asparagus and cherry tomatoes.

Nutritional Information (per serving):

- Calories: 370
- Protein: 30g
- Fat: 21g

- Carbohydrates: 10g
- Fiber: 3g
- Sugar: 5g

Cooking Time: 25 minutes
Serving Size: 4 servings

Recipe 3:

Grilled Pork Chops with Steamed Asparagus and Parmesan

Ingredients:

- 4 pork chops
- 1 pound asparagus, trimmed
- 2 tablespoons olive oil
- 2 cloves garlic, minced
- 1/4 cup grated Parmesan cheese
- Salt and pepper to taste

Instructions:

1. Preheat the grill to medium-high heat.
2. Rub the pork chops with 1 tablespoon of olive oil, minced garlic, salt, and pepper.

3. Grill the pork chops for about 5-7 minutes per side, or until the internal temperature reaches 145°F (63°C).
4. While the pork chops are grilling, steam the asparagus in a steamer basket over boiling water for about 5-7 minutes, or until tender.
5. Drizzle the steamed asparagus with the remaining tablespoon of olive oil and sprinkle with grated Parmesan cheese. Season with salt and pepper to taste.
6. Serve the grilled pork chops with the Parmesan-topped steamed asparagus.

Nutritional Information (per serving):

- Calories: 360
- Protein: 31g
- Fat: 21g
- Carbohydrates: 9g
- Fiber: 3g
- Sugar: 3g

Cooking Time: 25 minutes
Serving Size: 4 servings

Recipe 4:

Grilled Pork Chops with Steamed Asparagus and Lemon Zest

Ingredients:

- 4 pork chops
- 1 pound asparagus, trimmed
- 2 tablespoons olive oil
- 2 cloves garlic, minced
- 1 teaspoon lemon zest
- Salt and pepper to taste

Instructions:

1. Preheat the grill to medium-high heat.
2. Rub the pork chops with 1 tablespoon of olive oil, minced garlic, salt, and pepper.
3. Grill the pork chops for about 5-7 minutes per side, or until the internal temperature reaches 145°F (63°C).
4. While the pork chops are grilling, steam the asparagus in a steamer basket over boiling water for about 5-7 minutes, or until tender.

5. Drizzle the steamed asparagus with the remaining tablespoon of olive oil and sprinkle with lemon zest. Season with salt and pepper to taste.
6. Serve the grilled pork chops with the lemon-zested steamed asparagus.

Nutritional Information (per serving):

- Calories: 355
- Protein: 30g
- Fat: 20g
- Carbohydrates: 8g
- Fiber: 3g
- Sugar: 3g

Cooking Time: 25 minutes
Serving Size: 4 servings

CONCLUSION

Navigating the dietary needs of seniors with Stage 3 kidney disease is an essential aspect of managing their overall health and well-being. At this critical stage, the kidneys are moderately impaired, making it crucial to adopt a diet that supports kidney function while preventing further damage. A well-balanced, kidney-friendly diet can significantly slow disease progression, improve quality of life, and minimize the risk of complications.

A diet for seniors in Stage 3 kidney disease typically involves moderate protein intake, emphasizing high-quality sources to ensure essential amino acids are available without overburdening the kidneys. Managing sodium intake is equally important, as it helps control blood pressure and reduces fluid retention, both of which are critical for kidney health. Limiting foods high in phosphorus and potassium can also prevent imbalances that can lead to further complications.

Fostering a diet rich in fruits, vegetables, whole grains, and healthy fats, while being mindful of the specific restrictions and requirements, can help seniors maintain their energy levels, support their immune system, and promote overall health. It is also vital to stay hydrated with appropriate fluid intake, as guided by healthcare professionals.

Incorporating these dietary principles requires a collaborative approach, involving dietitians, healthcare providers, caregivers, and the seniors themselves. Education and support are key, ensuring that seniors understand the impact of their dietary choices and feel empowered to make adjustments that benefit their health. Regular monitoring and adjustments based on medical advice are crucial to respond to the changing needs of the kidneys and overall health status.

Ultimately, a carefully planned kidney disease diet for seniors in Stage 3 can make a profound difference. It can slow the progression of kidney disease, enhance quality of life, and provide a sense of control and well-being. By prioritizing nutrition and making informed dietary choices, seniors can navigate the challenges of Stage 3 kidney disease with greater resilience and hope for a better quality of life.

www.ingramcontent.com/pod-product-compliance
Lightning Source LLC
Chambersburg PA
CBHW071945210526
45479CB00002B/818